GAPS DIET COOKBOOK

Mary Dixon

TABLE OF CONTENT

CHAPTER ONE

Types, Causes and Symptoms of GAPS Disease

GAPS (**Gut and Psychology Syndrome**) is a term coined by Dr. Natasha Campbell-McBride, a neurologist and nutritionist, to describe a complex condition believed to originate in the gut and affect both physical and mental health.

It's important to note that GAPS is not recognized as a distinct medical diagnosis by mainstream medical authorities, and its concepts and treatments remain controversial.

Dr. Campbell-McBride's work primarily focuses on the gut-brain connection and suggests that imbalances in the gut flora can lead to various physical and psychological symptoms.

Here, we'll explore the types, potential causes, and symptoms associated with GAPS as described by proponents of this concept.

Types of GAPS:

1. Gut Dysbiosis: GAPS theory suggests that imbalances in the gut microbiome are at the core of the condition. It is believed to encompass several subtypes of GAPS:

- Gut Dysbiosis: An imbalance in the gut bacteria, where harmful microbes outnumber beneficial ones, leading to digestive issues and inflammation.
- Psychological GAPS: This subtype suggests a link between gut health and mental health conditions such as anxiety, depression, and autism spectrum disorders.
- Immune GAPS: Immune system dysfunction is believed to result from compromised gut health, leading to frequent infections and allergies.
- Autoimmune GAPS: GAPS proponents argue that autoimmune diseases can be triggered or exacerbated by a compromised gut lining, causing the immune system to attack the body's own tissues.

Causes of GAPS:

1. Diet: GAPS theory emphasizes the role of a poor diet high in processed foods, sugars, and antibiotics in disrupting the gut microbiome. Antibiotic use, in particular, can lead to imbalances in gut bacteria.

2. Environmental Factors: Exposure to environmental toxins, such as heavy metals, pesticides, and pollutants, is believed to contribute to gut health deterioration.

3. Stress: Chronic stress can affect the gut-brain axis, potentially leading to gut problems and mental health issues.

4. Genetics: Some proponents suggest a genetic predisposition to GAPS, meaning certain individuals may be more susceptible to gut-related issues.

Symptoms of GAPS:

The symptoms associated with GAPS are numerous and can vary from person to person.

These symptoms are often divided into physical and psychological categories:

Physical Symptoms:

1. Digestive Issues:

- Chronic diarrhea or constipation
- Abdominal pain and bloating

- Food intolerances and sensitivities

2. Skin Problems:

- Eczema and other skin rashes
- Acne
- Itchy skin

3. Immune System Dysfunction:

- Frequent infections
- Allergies and sensitivities

4. Autoimmune Conditions:

- Rheumatoid arthritis
- Hashimoto's thyroiditis
- Type 1 diabetes

5. Nutritional Deficiencies:

- Malabsorption issues leading to deficiencies in vitamins and minerals

Psychological Symptoms:

1. Anxiety

2. Depression

3. Attention deficit and hyperactivity (ADHD)

4. Autism spectrum disorders (ASD)

5. Behavioral problems in children

It's important to note that the concept of GAPS and its proposed causes and symptoms remain controversial in mainstream medicine.

While there is evidence supporting the role of the gut microbiome in health, the specific claims made by GAPS proponents are not universally accepted.

Individuals experiencing these symptoms should consult with healthcare professionals for a proper diagnosis and evidence-based treatment options.

GAPS Diet with Benefits

The GAPS (Gut and Psychology Syndrome) diet is a dietary protocol developed by Dr. Natasha Campbell-McBride to address gut health and its potential impact on various physical and psychological conditions.

It's important to note that while some individuals claim benefits from following the GAPS diet, it remains controversial and is not recognized as a mainstream medical treatment

If you are considering the GAPS diet, it's essential to consult with a healthcare professional, especially a registered dietitian or nutritionist, to ensure it's appropriate for your specific health needs and to monitor your progress.

Here are the general guidelines for following a GAPS diet:

1. Stages of the GAPS Diet:

The GAPS diet is typically divided into several stages, starting with the most restrictive and gradually allowing for more foods as gut healing progresses.

These stages are:

a. Introduction Stage: This is the most restrictive stage and consists of homemade bone broths, fermented foods, and well-cooked vegetables. It lasts for several weeks or even months, depending on individual needs.

b. Full GAPS Diet: Once the introduction stage is completed successfully, you can transition to the full GAPS diet. This stage includes a wider variety of foods, such as meats, fish, eggs, and some fruits and vegetables.

c. Customizing the Diet: Over time, individuals can customize the diet to suit their specific needs, reintroducing foods cautiously while monitoring their body's response.

2. Key Foods and Components:

- Bone Broth: Rich in amino acids and collagen, bone broth is a staple in the GAPS diet and supports gut healing.
- Probiotic-Rich Foods: Fermented foods like sauerkraut, kefir, and yogurt (if tolerated) are encouraged to promote a healthy gut microbiome.
- Animal Proteins: Organic meats, poultry, and fish are primary protein sources. These should be well-cooked and preferably sourced from grass-fed or pasture-raised animals.
- Healthy Fats: Include sources of healthy fats like avocado, coconut oil, and olive oil in your diet.
- Non-Starchy Vegetables: Focus on well-cooked, non-starchy vegetables, such as zucchini, carrots, and broccoli.
- Fruits: Initially, limit fruit intake to non-citrus, low-sugar options like berries and apples. As you progress, you can introduce more fruits.

- Nuts and Seeds: Some individuals may be able to tolerate small amounts of soaked and dehydrated nuts and seeds.
- Eggs: Eggs are generally allowed once the introduction stage is completed.

3. Foods to Avoid:

- Processed Foods: Eliminate processed and packaged foods, as they often contain additives, preservatives, and sugars that can be harmful to gut health.
- Grains and Gluten: Wheat, barley, rye, and other grains containing gluten are avoided on the GAPS diet.
- High Sugar Foods: Sugar, high-fructose corn syrup, and artificial sweeteners should be avoided.
- Starchy Vegetables: Limit starchy vegetables like potatoes until the full GAPS diet stage.
- Dairy: Dairy is eliminated during the initial stages, but some individuals may reintroduce dairy products like homemade yogurt or ghee later on.

4. Supplements and Lifestyle Factors:

- Probiotic supplements may be recommended to support the gut microbiome.

- Digestive enzymes and other supplements may be suggested by a healthcare professional.
- Reducing stress and getting adequate sleep are crucial for overall health and gut healing.

5. Individualized Approach: It's essential to understand that the GAPS diet should be individualized based on your specific health needs and symptoms. Some people may benefit from this approach, while others may not.

Always consult with a healthcare professional before making significant dietary changes, especially if you have underlying health conditions.

6. Monitoring and Evaluation: Regularly monitor your progress, symptoms, and overall well-being while following the GAPS diet. Adjust the diet as needed and seek professional guidance to ensure you are meeting your nutritional requirements.

Remember that the GAPS diet can be quite restrictive and may not be suitable for everyone. Always consult with a healthcare provider to determine the most appropriate approach for your health and nutritional needs.

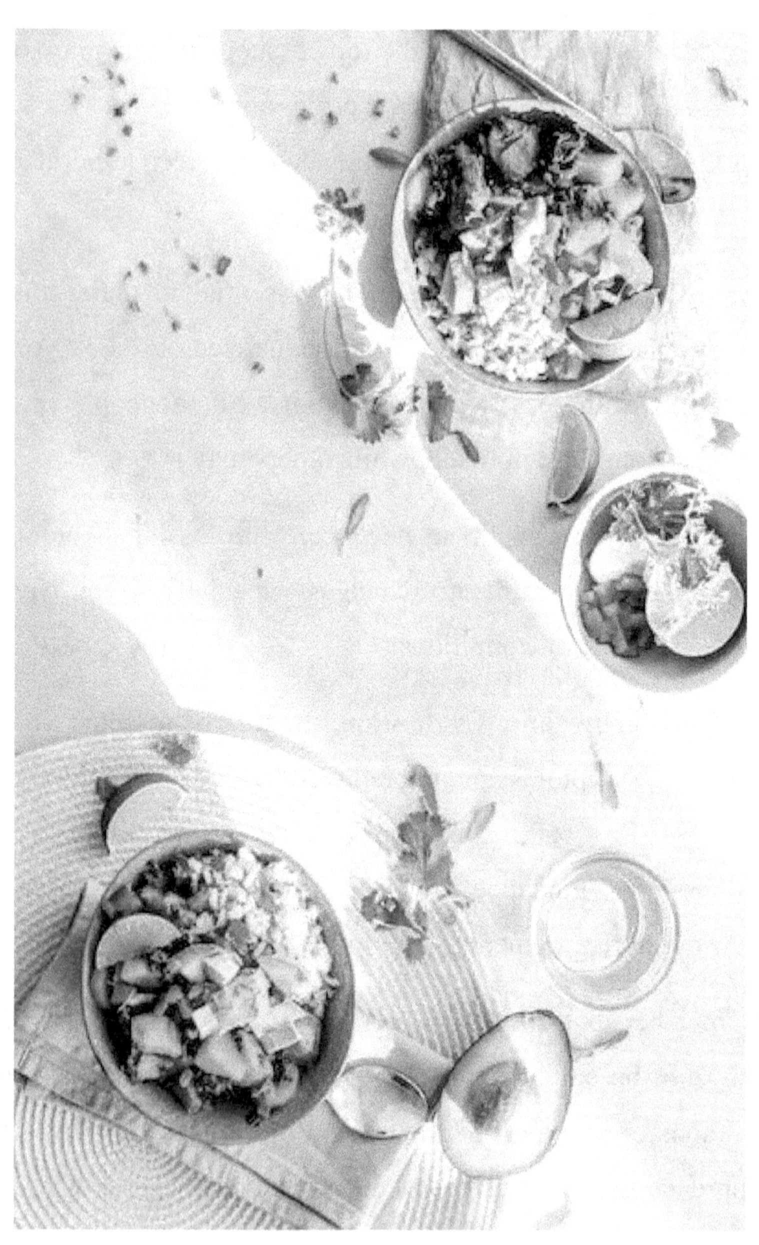

CHAPTER TWO

14-Day GAPS Diet Meal Plan

Creating a comprehensive 14-day GAPS (Gut and Psychology Syndrome) diet meal plan requires careful consideration of the diet's stages and the gradual introduction of foods.

Keep in mind that the GAPS diet is quite restrictive, so it's crucial to consult with a healthcare professional or registered dietitian before starting and to adapt the plan to your specific needs.

Below is a sample 14-day GAPS diet meal plan to give you an idea of how to structure your meals:

Day 1: Introduction Stage

- Breakfast: Homemade chicken broth with boiled carrots.
- Lunch: Steamed zucchini with ghee.
- Snack: Homemade yogurt (if tolerated).
- Dinner: Baked salmon with well-cooked broccoli.

Day 2: Introduction Stage

- Breakfast: Homemade beef broth with boiled squash.

- Lunch: Mashed cauliflower with homemade chicken broth.
- Snack: Fermented sauerkraut.
- Dinner: Roast chicken with butternut squash puree.

Day 3: Introduction Stage

- Breakfast: Homemade fish broth with steamed asparagus.
- Lunch: Pureed carrot soup with ghee.
- Snack: A small portion of boiled chicken.
- Dinner: Beef stew with well-cooked cabbage.

Day 4: Introduction Stage

- Breakfast: Homemade lamb broth with boiled cauliflower.
- Lunch: Pureed broccoli soup with ghee.
- Snack: Homemade yogurt with honey (if tolerated).
- Dinner: Pan-fried white fish with sautéed spinach.

Day 5: Introduction Stage

- Breakfast: Homemade turkey broth with boiled zucchini.
- Lunch: Mashed carrot and turnip with ghee.
- Snack: Fermented pickles.

- Dinner: Roast pork with steamed green beans.

Day 6: Transition to Full GAPS Diet

- Breakfast: Scrambled eggs with spinach cooked in coconut oil.
- Lunch: Grilled chicken breast with mixed greens and olive oil dressing.
- Snack: Avocado slices.
- Dinner: Baked cod with roasted Brussels sprouts.

Day 7: Full GAPS Diet

- Breakfast: Omelette with mushrooms and onions.
- Lunch: Beef stir-fry with broccoli and cauliflower rice.
- Snack: Homemade yogurt with berries (if tolerated).
- Dinner: Lemon herb roasted chicken with sautéed kale.

Day 8: Full GAPS Diet

- Breakfast: Smoked salmon with avocado and cucumber slices.
- Lunch: Turkey and vegetable soup with bone broth.
- Snack: Fermented carrots.
- Dinner: Grilled shrimp with roasted asparagus.

Day 9: Full GAPS Diet

- Breakfast: Greek yogurt with honey and almonds (if tolerated).
- Lunch: Beef and vegetable curry with cauliflower rice.
- Snack: Almond butter on celery sticks.
- Dinner: Baked lamb chops with garlic and rosemary, served with sautéed Swiss chard.

Day 10: Full GAPS Diet

- Breakfast: Scrambled eggs with diced tomatoes and basil.
- Lunch: Chicken and vegetable stir-fry with coconut aminos.
- Snack: Fermented cabbage.
- Dinner: Baked cod with a lemon dill sauce, accompanied by steamed broccoli.

Day 11: Full GAPS Diet

- Breakfast: Scrambled eggs with diced bell peppers and onions.
- Lunch: Pork tenderloin with a side of sautéed spinach and garlic.

- Snack: Mixed berries with a dollop of homemade yogurt (if tolerated).
- Dinner: Grilled shrimp skewers with a side of roasted Brussels sprouts and a lemon-garlic aioli.

Day 12: Full GAPS Diet

- Breakfast: Greek yogurt with honey and chopped almonds (if tolerated).
- Lunch: Beef and vegetable stir-fry with broccoli and cauliflower rice.
- Snack: Almond butter on cucumber slices.
- Dinner: Baked chicken thighs with a side of asparagus and a lemon herb sauce.

Day 13: Full GAPS Diet

- Breakfast: Scrambled eggs with diced tomatoes and fresh basil.
- Lunch: Turkey and vegetable soup with homemade bone broth.
- Snack: Fermented beet slices.
- Dinner: Baked salmon with a creamy dill sauce, served with sautéed Swiss chard.

Day 14: Full GAPS Diet

- Breakfast: Omelette with mushrooms, spinach, and onions.
- Lunch: Chicken breast with a side salad of mixed greens, cherry tomatoes, and an olive oil vinaigrette.
- Snack: A handful of mixed nuts (if tolerated).
- Dinner: Grilled lamb chops with roasted asparagus and a mint pesto.

As you progress through these days, feel free to continue introducing more variety into your diet, including different proteins, vegetables, and healthy fats.

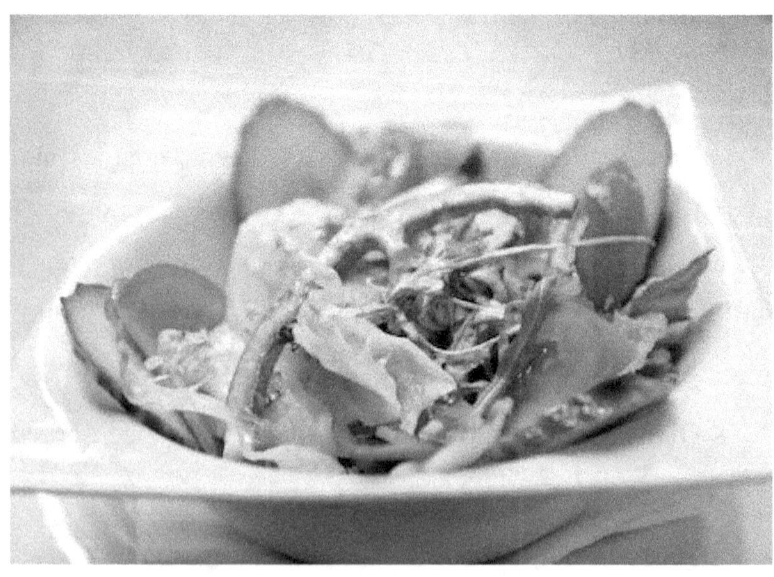

CHAPTER THREE

GAPS Diet Breakfast Recipes

Here are GAPS diet-friendly breakfast recipes with a short introduction, ingredients, instructions, and estimated cooking times.

These recipes are designed to support gut health and are free from grains, processed sugars, and other potentially irritating

Ingredients:

1. Scrambled Eggs with Spinach

Start your day with a protein-packed breakfast rich in nutrients.

Ingredients:

- 2 large eggs
- Handful of fresh spinach leaves
- Salt and pepper to taste
- Coconut oil or ghee for cooking

Instructions:

1. Whisk the eggs in a bowl and season with salt and pepper.

2. Heat coconut oil or ghee in a skillet over medium heat.

3. Add spinach leaves and sauté until wilted.

4. Pour in the beaten eggs and scramble until cooked to your liking.

Cooking Time: 5-7 minutes

2. Homemade Chicken Broth with Vegetables

A warm and nourishing option for gut healing.

Ingredients:

- 1 cup homemade chicken broth
- 1/2 cup diced carrots
- 1/2 cup diced zucchini
- Fresh parsley (optional)
- Salt and pepper to taste

Instructions:

1. Heat the chicken broth in a saucepan.

2. Add carrots and simmer until slightly tender.

3. Add zucchini and continue to simmer until all vegetables are cooked.

4. Season with salt and pepper, garnish with fresh parsley if desired.

Cooking Time: 10-15 minutes

3. Avocado and Smoked Salmon Salad

A satisfying breakfast with healthy fats and omega-3s.

Ingredients:

- 1 ripe avocado, sliced
- 2-3 slices of smoked salmon
- Lemon juice
- Fresh dill (optional)
- Salt and pepper to taste

Instructions:

1. Arrange avocado slices on a plate.

2. Top with smoked salmon.

3. Squeeze lemon juice over the dish and season with salt, pepper, and fresh dill.

Cooking Time: No cooking required

4. Homemade Yogurt with Berries

A probiotic-rich breakfast with the natural sweetness of berries.

Ingredients:

- 1 cup homemade yogurt
- Mixed berries (e.g., strawberries, blueberries, raspberries)
- Honey (optional, if tolerated)

Instructions:

1. Spoon homemade yogurt into a bowl.

2. Add a handful of mixed berries on top.

3. Drizzle with honey for sweetness if desired.

Cooking Time: No cooking required

5. Zucchini Fritters

A savory breakfast option that's both tasty and gut-friendly.

Ingredients:

- 2 medium zucchinis, grated and squeezed of excess moisture

- 2 eggs

- 2 tablespoons coconut flour

- Salt and pepper to taste

- Coconut oil for frying

Instructions:

1. In a bowl, mix grated zucchini, eggs, coconut flour, salt, and pepper.

2. Heat coconut oil in a skillet over medium-high heat.

3. Drop spoonfuls of the mixture into the skillet and flatten to form fritters.

4. Cook until golden brown on both sides.

Cooking Time: 15-20 minutes

6. Turkey and Vegetable Scramble

A protein-packed breakfast with a medley of colorful veggies.

Ingredients:

- Ground turkey

- Chopped bell peppers, onions, and spinach

- Coconut oil or ghee for cooking

- Salt and pepper to taste

Instructions:

1. Heat coconut oil or ghee in a skillet over medium heat.

2. Add ground turkey and cook until browned.

3. Add chopped vegetables and sauté until tender.

4. Season with salt and pepper.

Cooking Time: 15-20 minutes

7. Berry and Coconut Smoothie

A refreshing and nutrient-packed way to start your day.

Ingredients:

- 1/2 cup homemade yogurt
- Mixed berries
- Coconut milk (unsweetened)
- Honey (optional, if tolerated)
- Ice cubes

Instructions:

1. Blend yogurt, mixed berries, coconut milk, and ice cubes until smooth.

2. Add honey for sweetness if desired.

Cooking Time: No cooking required

8. Sausage and Vegetable Skillet

A hearty breakfast skillet loaded with flavor.

Ingredients:

- Sausage (look for preservative-free options)
- Chopped bell peppers, onions, and zucchini
- Coconut oil for cooking
- Salt and pepper to taste

Instructions:

1. Slice sausage into rounds.

2. Heat coconut oil in a skillet over medium heat.

3. Add sausage and cook until browned.

4. Add chopped vegetables and sauté until tender.

5. Season with salt and pepper.

Cooking Time: 15-20 minutes

9. Spinach and Bacon Omelette

A classic omelette with the goodness of spinach and bacon.

Ingredients:

- 2-3 eggs
- Fresh spinach leaves
- Cooked bacon bits (nitrate-free)
- Coconut oil or ghee for cooking
- Salt and pepper to taste

Instructions:

1. Whisk the eggs in a bowl and season with salt and pepper.

2. Heat coconut oil or ghee in a skillet over medium heat.

3. Add fresh spinach and sauté until wilted.

4. Pour in the beaten eggs and sprinkle with bacon bits. Cook until set and fold in half.

Cooking Time: 5-7 minutes

10. Coconut Flour Pancakes

Fluffy and grain-free pancakes for a special morning treat.

Ingredients:

- 1/4 cup coconut flour
- 2 eggs
- 1/4 cup homemade yogurt
- 1/4 cup unsweetened coconut milk
- 1/2 teaspoon baking soda
- Coconut oil for cooking
- Fresh berries for topping

Instructions:

1. In a bowl, whisk together coconut flour, eggs, yogurt, coconut milk, and baking soda until well combined.

2. Heat coconut oil in a skillet over medium heat.

3. Pour small portions of the batter onto the skillet to form pancakes.

4. Cook until bubbles form on the surface, then flip and cook until golden brown.

5. Top with fresh berries.

Cooking Time: 10-15 minutes

GAPS Diet Lunch Recipes

1. Homemade Chicken Soup

A comforting and nourishing soup that's perfect for lunch.

Ingredients:

- Homemade chicken broth
- Cooked chicken pieces
- Carrots, celery, and onions, diced
- Salt and pepper to taste
- Fresh parsley (optional)

Instructions:

1. Heat homemade chicken broth in a pot.

2. Add cooked chicken pieces, diced vegetables, and season with salt and pepper.

3. Simmer until the vegetables are tender.

4. Garnish with fresh parsley if desired.

Cooking Time: 15-20 minutes

2. Beef and Vegetable Stir-Fry

A flavorful and satisfying stir-fry loaded with veggies.

Ingredients:

- Sliced beef (e.g., sirloin or flank steak)
- Chopped broccoli, bell peppers, and zucchini
- Coconut aminos for seasoning
- Coconut oil for cooking
- Garlic and ginger (optional)

Instructions:

1. Heat coconut oil in a skillet over high heat.

2. Stir-fry beef until browned. Remove from the skillet.

3. Add more coconut oil if needed and stir-fry chopped vegetables.

4. Return the beef to the skillet, add coconut aminos, and season with garlic and ginger if desired.

Cooking Time: 15-20 minutes

3. Turkey and Vegetable Soup

A wholesome and protein-rich soup with a medley of vegetables.

Ingredients:

- Ground turkey
- Chopped carrots, zucchini, and spinach
- Homemade turkey or chicken broth
- Salt and pepper to taste

Instructions:

1. In a pot, brown ground turkey.

2. Add chopped vegetables and homemade broth.

3. Season with salt and pepper and simmer until vegetables are tender.

Cooking Time: 20-25 minutes

4. Baked Salmon with Lemon-Dill Sauce

A simple and flavorful way to enjoy salmon for lunch.

Ingredients:

- Salmon fillet
- Fresh lemon juice
- Fresh dill
- Salt and pepper to taste

Instructions:

1. Preheat the oven to 375°F (190°C).

2. Place salmon on a baking sheet.

3. Drizzle with lemon juice, sprinkle with fresh dill, salt, and pepper.

4. Bake until the salmon flakes easily with a fork.

Cooking Time: 15-20 minutes

5. Turkey and Avocado Lettuce Wraps

A light and nutritious lunch option.

Ingredients:

- Ground turkey
- Lettuce leaves for wrapping
- Avocado slices
- Chopped tomatoes and red onion
- Fresh cilantro (optional)
- Salt and pepper to taste

Instructions:

1. Brown ground turkey in a skillet.

2. Season with salt and pepper.

3. Arrange lettuce leaves, turkey, avocado, tomatoes, and red onion.

4. Garnish with fresh cilantro if desired.

Cooking Time: 15 minutes

6. Chicken and Vegetable Salad

A fresh and vibrant salad with grilled chicken.

Ingredients:

- Grilled chicken breast, sliced
- Mixed greens (e.g., lettuce, spinach)
- Cherry tomatoes
- Cucumber slices
- Olive oil and balsamic vinegar for dressing
- Salt and pepper to taste

Instructions:

1. Arrange mixed greens on a plate.

2. Top with grilled chicken, cherry tomatoes, and cucumber slices.

3. Drizzle with olive oil and balsamic vinegar.

4. Season with salt and pepper.

Cooking Time: Varies (assuming chicken is pre-cooked)

7. Homemade Vegetable Soup

A versatile and nutrient-rich soup with a variety of vegetables.

Ingredients:

- Homemade vegetable broth
- Assorted vegetables (e.g., carrots, celery, cauliflower)
- Fresh herbs (e.g., thyme, rosemary)
- Salt and pepper to taste

Instructions:

1. Heat homemade vegetable broth in a pot.

2. Add diced vegetables and fresh herbs.

3. Season with salt and pepper.

4. Simmer until vegetables are tender.

Cooking Time: 20-25 minutes

8. Beef and Spinach Salad

A hearty salad with sautéed beef and nutrient-packed spinach.

Ingredients:

- Sliced beef (e.g., sirloin)
- Fresh spinach leaves
- Chopped red onion
- Sliced mushrooms
- Olive oil and lemon juice for dressing
- Salt and pepper to taste

Instructions:

1. Sauté sliced beef in a skillet until browned.

2. In a large bowl, combine fresh spinach, red onion, and sliced mushrooms.

3. Drizzle with olive oil and lemon juice.

4. Add the cooked beef and season with salt and pepper.

Cooking Time: 10-15 minutes

9. Shrimp and Avocado Salad

A light and refreshing salad with shrimp and creamy avocado.

Ingredients:

-   Cooked shrimp
-   Avocado, diced
-   Chopped cucumber and cherry tomatoes
-   Fresh cilantro (optional)
-   Olive oil and lime juice for dressing
-   Salt and pepper to taste

Instructions:

1. Combine cooked shrimp, diced avocado, chopped cucumber, and cherry tomatoes in a bowl.

2. Drizzle with olive oil and lime juice.

3. Garnish with fresh cilantro if desired.

4. Season with salt and pepper.

Cooking Time: Varies (assuming shrimp is pre-cooked)

10. Baked Chicken Thighs with Roasted Vegetables

A satisfying and complete meal with baked chicken and roasted vegetables.

Ingredients:

- Chicken thighs
- Assorted vegetables (e.g., carrots, Brussels sprouts, bell peppers)
- Olive oil and herbs (e.g., rosemary, thyme)
- Salt and pepper to taste

Instructions:

1. Preheat the oven to 375°F (190°C).

2. Arrange chicken thighs and vegetables on a baking sheet.

3. Drizzle with olive oil, sprinkle with herbs, salt, and pepper.

4. Bake until chicken is cooked through and vegetables are tender.

Cooking Time: 30-35 minutes

CHAPTER FOUR

GAPS Diet Dinner Recipes

1. Lemon Herb Roasted Chicken

A flavorful and juicy roasted chicken with a zesty twist.

Ingredients:

- Whole chicken
- Fresh lemon juice and zest
- Fresh herbs (e.g., rosemary, thyme)
- Salt and pepper to taste

Instructions:

1. Preheat the oven to 375°F (190°C).

2. Rub the chicken with lemon juice, zest, fresh herbs, salt, and pepper.

3. Roast in the oven until the chicken reaches a safe internal temperature.

Cooking Time: Approximately 1.5 hours (varies based on the size of the chicken)

2. Beef and Vegetable Stew

A hearty stew filled with tender beef and a medley of vegetables.

Ingredients:

- Stewing beef
- Chopped carrots, celery, and onions
- Homemade beef broth
- Fresh herbs (e.g., thyme, bay leaves)
- Salt and pepper to taste

Instructions:

1. In a large pot, brown the stewing beef.

2. Add chopped vegetables, homemade beef broth, fresh herbs, salt, and pepper.

3. Simmer until the beef is tender and the flavors meld.

Cooking Time: Approximately 2 hours

3. Grilled Salmon with Garlic and Dill

A simple and healthy dinner with grilled salmon and aromatic garlic and dill.

Ingredients:

- Salmon fillets
- Fresh garlic, minced
- Fresh dill, chopped
- Lemon juice
- Salt and pepper to taste

Instructions:

1. Preheat the grill to medium-high heat.

2. Season salmon fillets with minced garlic, chopped dill, lemon juice, salt, and pepper.

3. Grill until salmon flakes easily with a fork.

Cooking Time: 10-15 minutes

4. Baked Turkey Meatballs with Zucchini Noodles

A low-carb and savory dinner option with turkey meatballs and zucchini noodles.

Ingredients:

- Ground turkey
- Almond flour (as a binder)

- Chopped garlic and onion
- Zucchini, spiralized into noodles
- Olive oil for cooking
- Salt and pepper to taste

Instructions:

1. Mix ground turkey, almond flour, chopped garlic, chopped onion, salt, and pepper to form meatballs.

2. Bake meatballs in the oven until cooked through.

3. Sauté zucchini noodles in olive oil until tender.

4. Serve meatballs over the zucchini noodles.

Cooking Time: 25-30 minutes

5. Lemon Garlic Shrimp Stir-Fry

A quick and flavorful stir-fry with shrimp and fresh lemon and garlic.

Ingredients:

- Shrimp
- Chopped broccoli, bell peppers, and snow peas
- Fresh lemon juice and zest
- Minced garlic

- Coconut oil for cooking

- Salt and pepper to taste

Instructions:

1. Heat coconut oil in a skillet over high heat.

2. Sauté shrimp until pink and cooked.

3. Remove shrimp and set aside.

4. In the same skillet, sauté chopped vegetables, minced garlic, lemon juice, and zest.

5. Return the cooked shrimp to the skillet and toss until heated through.

Cooking Time: 15-20 minutes

6. Roast Pork with Cabbage and Apples

A delightful combination of roast pork, caramelized apples, and tender cabbage.

Ingredients:

- Pork roast (e.g., loin or shoulder)

- Sliced apples

- Chopped cabbage

- Cinnamon (optional)
- Salt and pepper to taste

Instructions:

1. Preheat the oven to 375°F (190°C).

2. Season the pork roast with salt, pepper, and optional cinnamon.

3. Roast the pork in the oven until it reaches a safe internal temperature.

4. In a separate skillet, sauté sliced apples and chopped cabbage until tender and caramelized.

Cooking Time: Approximately 1.5-2 hours (varies based on pork size)

7. Lemon Herb Grilled Chicken Thighs

A delicious and herb-infused grilled chicken dinner.

Ingredients:

- Chicken thighs
- Fresh lemon juice and zest
- Chopped fresh herbs (e.g., rosemary, thyme)
- Olive oil

\-   Salt and pepper to taste

Instructions:

1. Preheat the grill to medium-high heat.

2. Season chicken thighs with fresh lemon juice, zest, chopped herbs, olive oil, salt, and pepper.

3. Grill until chicken reaches a safe internal temperature.

Cooking Time: 15-20 minutes

8. Beef and Cauliflower Rice Stir-Fry

A low-carb stir-fry with tender beef and cauliflower rice.

Ingredients:

-   Sliced beef (e.g., flank steak)
-   Cauliflower, grated into "rice"
-   Chopped bell peppers and snap peas
-   Coconut aminos for seasoning
-   Coconut oil for cooking
-   Salt and pepper to taste

Instructions:

1. Heat coconut oil in a skillet over high heat.

2. Sauté sliced beef until browned.

3. Remove beef and set aside.

4. In the same skillet, stir-fry cauliflower rice, chopped vegetables, and coconut aminos.

5. Return the cooked beef to the skillet and toss until heated through.

Cooking Time: 20-25 minutes

9. Chicken and Vegetable Curry

A flavorful curry with tender chicken and an array of vegetables.

Ingredients:

- Chicken breast, diced
- Chopped bell peppers, zucchini, and carrots
- Curry spice blend (GAPS-friendly)
- Coconut milk (unsweetened)
- Coconut oil for cooking
- Salt and pepper to taste

Instructions:

1. In a skillet, heat coconut oil over medium heat.

2. Sauté diced chicken until browned.

3. Remove chicken and set aside.

4. In the same skillet, stir-fry chopped vegetables and curry spice blend.

5. Return the cooked chicken to the skillet and add coconut milk.

6. Simmer until the chicken is cooked through and the sauce thickens.

Cooking Time: 20-25 minutes

10. Herb-Crusted Baked White Fish

A light and flavorful dinner featuring baked white fish with fresh herbs.

Ingredients:

- White fish fillets (e.g., cod, haddock)
- Chopped fresh herbs (e.g., parsley, chives)
- Lemon juice and zest
- Olive oil
- Salt and pepper to taste

Instructions:

1. Preheat the oven to 375°F (190°C).

2. Season fish fillets with fresh herbs, lemon juice, zest, olive oil, salt, and pepper.

3. Bake in the oven until the fish flakes easily with a fork.

Cooking Time: 15-20 minutes

These GAPS diet dinner recipes offer a range of flavors and ingredients to keep your meals both delicious and supportive of gut health. Adjust portion sizes and ingredients to meet your specific dietary needs and

 preferences. Enjoy your nutritious and satisfying dinners!

GAPS Diet Snack Recipes

1. Fermented Carrot Sticks

A crunchy and probiotic-rich snack for gut health.

Ingredients:

- Fresh carrots, peeled and cut into sticks
- Sea salt
- Filtered water

Instructions:

1. Place carrot sticks in a glass jar.

2. Dissolve sea salt in filtered water to create a brine.

3. Pour the brine over the carrots until they are fully submerged.

4. Cover the jar with a lid and allow it to ferment at room temperature for a few days.

5. Once fermented to your liking, refrigerate and enjoy.

Preparation Time: 10 minutes (plus fermentation time)

2. Homemade Sauerkraut

A classic fermented snack packed with probiotics.

Ingredients:

- Cabbage, thinly sliced
- Sea salt

Instructions:

1. Massage sea salt into the thinly sliced cabbage until it starts releasing liquid.

2. Pack the cabbage tightly into a glass jar.

3. Ensure the cabbage is submerged in its liquid.

4. Cover the jar with a lid and let it ferment at room temperature for several days to weeks, depending on your taste preference.

5. Refrigerate after fermentation is complete.

Preparation Time: 20-30 minutes (plus fermentation time)

3. Almond Butter on Celery Sticks

A quick and nutritious snack with healthy fats and fiber.

Ingredients:

- Fresh celery sticks
- Homemade or store-bought almond butter (check for GAPS-compliant options)

Instructions:

1. Spread almond butter onto celery sticks.

2. Enjoy as a crunchy and satisfying snack.

Preparation Time: 5 minutes

4. Homemade Coconut Milk Yogurt

A dairy-free yogurt option rich in probiotics.

Ingredients:

- Fresh coconut milk (from mature coconuts)
- Probiotic capsules (GAPS-friendly strains)
- Raw honey (optional, if tolerated)

Instructions:

1. Blend fresh coconut meat and water to make coconut milk.

2. Mix coconut milk with probiotic capsules in a glass jar.

3. Cover the jar with a cloth and secure it with a rubber band.

4. Allow it to ferment at room temperature for 12-24 hours.

5. Refrigerate and sweeten with raw honey if desired before serving.

Preparation Time: 15-20 minutes (plus fermentation time)

5. Guacamole with Vegetable Sticks

A creamy and nutrient-rich dip with colorful vegetable sticks.

Ingredients:

- Ripe avocados
- Lime juice
- Chopped tomatoes, onions, and cilantro (optional)
- Salt and pepper to taste
- Fresh vegetable sticks (e.g., cucumber, bell peppers)

Instructions:

1. Mash ripe avocados and mix with lime juice.

2. Add chopped tomatoes, onions, cilantro, salt, and pepper if desired.

3. Serve with fresh vegetable sticks for dipping.

Preparation Time: 10-15 minutes

6. Fermented Pickles

A tangy and probiotic snack made from cucumbers.

Ingredients:

- Fresh cucumbers
- Fresh dill
- Garlic cloves
- Sea salt

- Filtered water

Instructions:

1. Pack cucumbers, fresh dill, and garlic cloves into a glass jar.

2. Dissolve sea salt in filtered water to create a brine.

3. Pour the brine over the cucumbers until they are fully submerged.

4. Cover the jar with a lid and let it ferment at room temperature for several days.

5. Once fermented to your liking, refrigerate and enjoy.

Preparation Time: 15-20 minutes (plus fermentation time)

7. Berry and Coconut Smoothie

A refreshing and antioxidant-rich snack.

Ingredients:

- Homemade yogurt
- Mixed berries (e.g., strawberries, blueberries, raspberries)
- Unsweetened coconut milk

- Raw honey (optional, if tolerated)

- Ice cubes

Instructions:

1. Blend homemade yogurt, mixed berries, coconut milk, raw honey, and ice cubes until smooth.

2. Adjust sweetness to taste with raw honey if desired.

Preparation Time: 5 minutes

8. Fermented Beet Slices

A unique and probiotic-packed snack with a vibrant color.

Ingredients:

- Fresh beets, peeled and thinly sliced

- Sea salt

- Filtered water

Instructions:

1. Place beet slices in a glass jar.

2. Dissolve sea salt in filtered water to create a brine.

3. Pour the brine over the beet slices until they are fully submerged.

4. Cover the jar with a lid and let it ferment at room temperature for several days.

5. Once fermented to your liking, refrigerate and enjoy.

Preparation Time: 10 minutes (plus fermentation time)

9. Coconut and Berry Parfait

A layered snack with coconut and mixed berries.

Ingredients:

- Homemade coconut yogurt
- Mixed berries (e.g., raspberries, blackberries)
- Raw honey (optional, if tolerated)
- Chopped nuts (e.g., almonds, walnuts) (optional)

Instructions:

1. Layer homemade coconut yogurt, mixed berries, and chopped nuts in a glass.

2. Drizzle with raw honey if desired.

Preparation Time: 5 minutes

10. Almond Flour Crackers

A crunchy and grain-free cracker option for snacking.

Ingredients:

- Almond flour
- Egg
- Coconut oil
- Salt and herbs (e.g., rosemary, thyme) (optional)

Instructions:

1. Mix almond flour, egg, coconut oil, salt, and optional herbs in a bowl to form a dough.

2. Roll out the dough and cut into cracker-sized pieces.

3. Bake in the oven until golden brown and crispy.

Preparation Time: 20-25 minutes

These GAPS diet snack recipes offer a variety of options to keep your snacking both delicious and gut-healthy. Adjust ingredients to meet your specific dietary needs and preferences. Enjoy your nutritious and satisfying snacks!

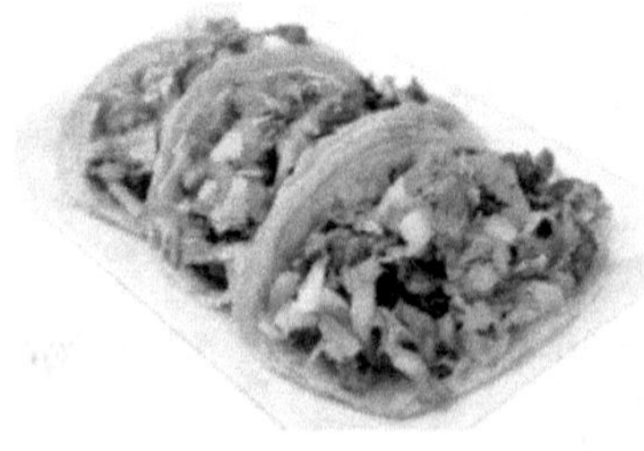

CONCLUSION

The Gut and Psychology Syndrome (GAPS) diet is a therapeutic and holistic approach to improving gut health, with far-reaching implications for overall well-being.

This diet places a strong emphasis on the connection between the gut and various physical and mental health conditions, highlighting the pivotal role that a healthy gut microbiome plays in our overall health.

The GAPS diet is structured in a way that promotes the healing of the gut lining, reduces inflammation, and supports the restoration of a balanced and diverse gut microbiota.

It achieves this by eliminating certain foods that can exacerbate gut issues, such as processed sugars, grains, and certain dairy products, while encouraging the consumption of nutrient-dense, whole foods like homemade broths, fermented foods, and organic vegetables.

This dietary approach is divided into stages, allowing individuals to gradually reintroduce foods as their gut health improves.

One of the notable strengths of the GAPS diet is its adaptability. It can be tailored to the specific needs of individuals with varying degrees of gut dysfunction, making it a valuable option for those dealing with conditions like irritable bowel syndrome (IBS), autoimmune diseases, autism spectrum disorders, and more.

However, it is crucial for anyone considering the GAPS diet to seek guidance from a healthcare professional or registered dietitian to ensure that it is appropriate for their unique circumstances.

The GAPS diet's potential benefits extend beyond gut health. Many individuals have reported improvements in symptoms related to mental health, allergies, skin conditions, and autoimmune disorders after following the diet.

While scientific research on the GAPS diet is ongoing, these anecdotal success stories highlight its promising role in enhancing overall quality of life.

It's important to acknowledge that the GAPS diet is not a one-size-fits-all solution, and its restrictive nature can pose challenges for some individuals. Moreover, it requires dedication and careful meal planning.

www.ingramcontent.com/pod-product-compliance
Lightning Source LLC
Chambersburg PA
CBHW071105260726

48661CB00006B/2479